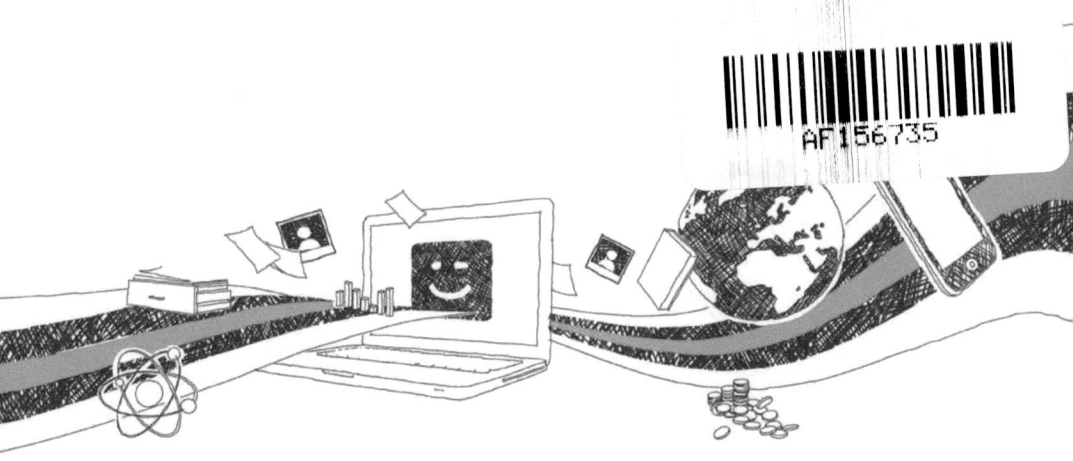
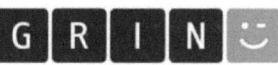

Imprint:

Copyright © 2017 GRIN Verlag, Open Publishing GmbH
Print and binding: Books on Demand GmbH, Norderstedt Germany
ISBN: 9783668478824

This book at GRIN:

http://www.grin.com/en/e-book/366629/review-of-lumpy-skin-disease-and-its-economic-impacts-in-ethiopia

Ahmed Farah

Review of Lumpy Skin Disease and Its Economic Impacts in Ethiopia

GRIN Publishing

GRIN - Your knowledge has value

Since its foundation in 1998, GRIN has specialized in publishing academic texts by students, college teachers and other academics as e-book and printed book. The website www.grin.com is an ideal platform for presenting term papers, final papers, scientific essays, dissertations and specialist books.

Visit us on the internet:

http://www.grin.com/

http://www.facebook.com/grincom

http://www.twitter.com/grin_com

REVIEW ON LUMPY SKIN DISEASE AND ITS ECONOMIC IMPACTS IN ETHIOPIA

By

Ahmed Ali   Farah Gumbe

A paper submitted to the College of Veterinary Medicine for the Course of Senior Seminar.

Mekelle University, College of Veterinary Medicine

March, 2017

Mekelle, Ethiopia

Table of Contents

ACKNOWLEDGEMENTS

All thanks are due to Allah, the owner of universe, who without his guidance will not be possible to take any step forward.

I wish to express my sincere thanks to my advisor, Dr. Equebaher Kassye, for his valuable constructive, advice, overall intellectual guidance, comments, suggestions and provision of literature materials.

I am deeply indebted thanks to my beloved family for all of their support whose without their generous financial and moral support will not be possible for me to attain my long lasting goals.

Last but not least, I wish thanks my beloved tutors, administrators and other supportive staff of Mekelle University, College of Veterinary Medicine; I will keep in mind the time we took together here in Mekelle University as whole of family and friends.

LIST OF TABLES

LIST OF FIGURES

LIST OF ABBREVIATIONS

AGID	Agar gel immunodiffusion
CSA	Central Statistics Authority
ELISA	Enzyme linked immune sorbent assay
FAO	World Food Organization
CSA	Central Statistics Authority
GTPV	Goat pox virus
LSDV	Lumpy skin disease virus
MoARD	Ministry of Agriculture and Rural Development
NVI	National Veterinary Institute
KS-1	Kenyan sheep pox strain 1
OIE	Office International des Epizooties, World Animal Health
PCR	Polymerase Chain Reaction
SNNPR	Southern nation nationalities and peoples region
SPPV	Sheep pox virus
USD	United States of Americas" Dollar
VNT	Virus neutralization test
CaPV	Capripoxviruses
DNA	Deoxyribonucleic cid
DsDNA	Double stranded Deoxyribonucleic
GDP	Gross Domestic product
Kbp	Kilo base pair
SGPV	Sheep and Goat Pox Virus

SUMMARY

Lumpy skin disease (LSD) is among the most economically significant viral diseases of cattle caused by Neethling virus prototype strain classified in the genus *Capripoxvirus* of family *Poxviridae*. The disease is characterized by fever, enlarged lymph nodes, firm and circumscribed nodules in the skin and nodules are particularly noticeable in the hairless areas. Lumpy skin disease is currently endemic in most Sub-Saharan African countries and subsequently spread to Middle East, Asia and to Europe countries. It is economically devastating viral diseases which cause several financial problems in livestock industries as a result of significant milk yield loss, infertility, abortion, trade limitation and sometimes death in most African countries including Ethiopia. In Ethiopia lumpy skin disease was first observed in the northwestern part of the country (southwest of Lake Tana) in 1983. It is now spread to almost all regions and agro-ecological zones of the country. Major epidemic outbreak of LSD has been documented in different regions of Ethiopia at different time period. From 2007 to 2011 a total of 1352 disease outbreaks of LSD have been documented. The highest outbreak was registered in Oromiya region and the lowest in Afar region. All breeds and age group, both sex are susceptible however, *Bos Taurus* are particularly more susceptible to clinical disease than *Bos indicus*. The various agro climatic conditions, introduction of new animals to the herd and the presence communal watering bodies are regard as major risk factors that would facilitate the spread of outbreaks in diverse localities. LSD is transmitted by mechanical vector insects and also wildlife plays a potential role in its maintenance. And could be diagnosed using appropriate serological and molecular techniques. The herd-level LSD prevalence is significantly higher in the midland agro-climate than in lowland and highland agro-climate zones due to abundance of speculated mechanical vector insects. Currently Effective control measures of this disease is achieved through mass vaccination, import restrictions on livestock and their products, control of vectors and quarantine station. Furthermore, culling of infected animals is also optional method.

Key Words: Bovine, Economic, Ethiopia, Infection, LSD.

1. INTRODUCTION

Livestock production constitutes one of the principal means of achieving improved living standards in many regions of the developing world (Anon, 2009). The livestock sector globally is highly dynamic, contributes 40% of the global value of agricultural output and support the livelihoods and food security of almost a billion people (Thornton, 2010). In many developing countries (In Sub-Saharan African countries), livestock keeping is a multifunctional activity and plays a crucial role both in national economies and the livelihood of rural communities, (FAO, 2009).

Ethiopia basically comprises an agrarian society; the socio-economic activities of about 85% of the population are based on farming and animal husbandry (RGBE, 2014). Ethiopia has the most abundant livestock population in Africa with the estimated domestic animal number of 57.83 million and cattle population is estimated to be 28.89 million (CSA, 2016).

Consequently Ethiopia livestock production is an integral part of the agricultural system. The livestock sub sector accounts for 40% of the agricultural gross domestic product (GDP) and 20% of the total GDP without considering other contribution like traction power, fertilizing and mean of transport (Gebreegziabhare, 2010).

Diseases are an important cause of reduced productivity of meat and milk as well as draft, hides and dung fuel. Lumpy skin disease (LSD) is among the most economically significant viral emerging diseases which is characterized by high fever, enlarged lymph nodes, firm, and circumscribed nodules (OIE, 2010). It is a disease with a high morbidity and low mortality rate and affects cattle of all ages and breeds. It causes high significant economic losses as a result of reduced milk production, beef loss and draft power loss, abortion, infertility, loss of condition and damage to the hide (CFSPH, 2008). Regarded to the office international des epizootics consider LSD as list A" disease that has the potential for rapid spread with ability to cause serious economic loss (RGBE, 2014).

LSD is currently endemic in most African continent and has recently spread out of Africa into the Middle East in additional to Europe countries (Tuppurinen and Oura, 2011). It becomes an important threat to livestock and dairy industry in the Middle East and Africa (Kumar, 2011). Despite it is transboundary disease, causes international ban on the trade of livestock and their products (Vorster and Mapham, 2008). Lumpy skin disease has a different geographical distribution from that of sheep- and goat-pox, suggesting that cattle strains of capripoxvirus do not infect or transmit between sheep and goats (Ahmed and Kawther, 2008).

In Ethiopia lumpy skin disease was first observed in the northwestern part of the country (southwest of Lake Tana) in 1983 (Mebratu et al., 1984). It is now spread to almost all regions and agro-ecological zones of the country. Vaccination is classically used to control outbreaks whenever they occur. Because of the wide distribution of the disease and the size and structure of the cattle population in Ethiopia. Major epidemic outbreak of LSD occurred in different regions of in different years Ethiopia like Amhara and W/ Oromiya Regions in 2000/2001, Oromiya and SNNP regions in 2003/2004 and Tigray, Amhara and Benishangul regions in 2006/2007 (Gari et al., 2010).

The most effective method of transmission is mechanically through biting flies. The incidence of LSD occurrence is high during wet seasons when biting-fly populations are abundant and it decreases or ceases during the dry season. Direct transmission can also occur between infected animals, but such transmission is rare and of low epidemiological significance (OIE, 2015b). The control measure of LSD can be achieved through vaccination and restriction of animal movement (Gari et al., 2012). Given that LSD is the one of the most economically important livestock disease in the country.

Therefore, the objectives of this Paper are to review on Lumpy skin disease and its economic impacts in Ethiopia.

2. LUMPY SKIN DISEASE

2.1. Etiology

LSDV is grouped under the family of *poxviridae*. The family *Poxviridae* is subdivided into two subfamilies: *Chordopoxvirinae* (poxviruses of vertebrates) and *Entomopoxvirinae* (poxviruses of insects). Lumpy skin disease virus (LSDV) belongs to the genus *Capripoxvirus and* the subfamily *Chordopoxvirinae*. There is only one serotype of LSDV which is prototype strain of LSDV is the Neethling virus and it is closely related antigenically to sheep and goat poxvirus and can be distinguished by routine virus neutralization or other serological tests. The LSDV primarily affects cattle but can affect sheep and goats, experimentally. Lumpy skin disease virus will grow in tissue culture of bovine, ovine or caprine origin, although maximum yield is obtained using lamb testis cells (Gelaye *et al.,* 2015). The members of this family are among the largest of all viruses. It is an envelope, Linear ovoid shape with a molecular brick shaped or ovoid virions measuring 220-450 nanometer (nm) by 140-266nm (Fig. 1). LSDV has ds DNA genome of about 151kb (Yehuda *et al.*, 2011).

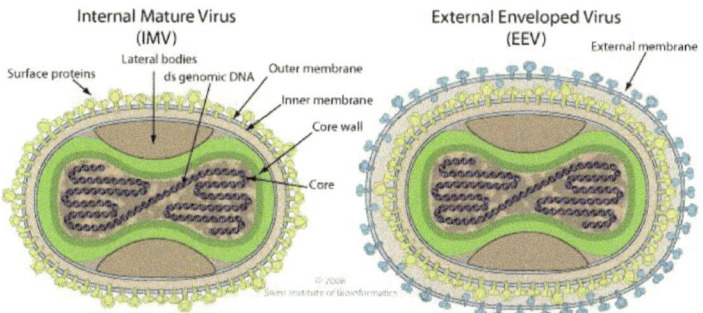

Figure 1: Morphological structure LSDV. Source (Lefèvre and Gourreau, 2010)

3

2. 2.Epidemiology

2.2.1. Geographical Distribution

Lumpy skin disease has a different geographical distribution (OIE, 2010). The disease was first observed in 1929 in Zambia. Initially, it was considered to be the result either of poisoning or a hypersensitivity to insect bites because at that time was it the year when populations of biting insects were greatest (Bagla, 2008). Between 1943 and 1945, cases occurred in Botswana, Zimbabwe (Southern Rhodesia) and the Republic of South Africa. The infectious nature of the disease was recognized at this time (OIE, 2008). The global distribution of LSD is presented in (Fi. 2) below.

LSD was restricted to countries in sub-Saharan Africa from 1929 to 1986 and it's endemic in most African countries including Madagascar. This Followed by reports of the virus in the Middle East Since 2012 LSD has been spreading on an unusually large scale throughout Middle Eastern countries as subsequently years was reported from Oman, Yemen, Israel, Kuwait, Bahrain, Egypt, Iran, Saudi Arabia Lebanon, Jordan, and in United Arab Emerate, (Zeynalova *et al.*, 2016).

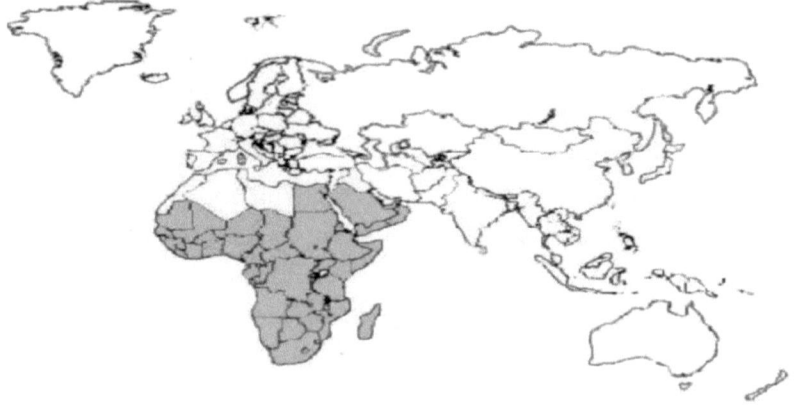

Figure 2: Global Distribution of lumpy skin disease in the World (2012).

Source: OIE. (2009).

Note: The shaded area shows LSD positive countries.   Source: http://www.epizone-eu.net/publicdocs/animal diseases/website LSD.

In Ethiopia LSD was spread to almost all the regions and agro ecological zones. While the large distribution of the disease and the size and structure of the cattle population (Gari et al., 2010). The data investigations from the national disease outbreak report database during the period 2000-2009 showed that major epidemic outbreaks of LSD occurred in 2000/2001 in the northern parts of the country in Amhara and West Oromia regions. Then it extended to the central and the southern parts of the country, in 2003 and 2004 covering large parts of Oromia and Southern Nation, Nationalities and Peoples (SNNP) regions. In 2006 and 2007 another extensive outbreak reappeared in Tigray, Amhara and Benishangul regions in the northern and north-western parts of the country. Therefore, from 2007 up to 2009 the outbreak number progressively increased in Oromia Region situated in the central part of the country while it seemed to be gradually decreasing in the northern part of the country including Tigray, Amhara and Benishangul regions (Gari, 2011).

According to 2010 annual report of Ministry of Agriculture, Animal and plant health regulatory directorate in the department of epidemiology prevalence of the disease in different regional state of the country shows us; 1.63%, 0.49%, 5.2%, 2.69%, 0.37%, 0.7%, and 3.8% in Addis Abeba, Amhara, Gambela, Oromia, SNNP, Somali and Tigray regions respectively. The 2011 annual report shows prevalence of; 0.36%, 1.13%, 0.22%, 0.65%, 0.24% and 0.30% in Amhara, Gambela, Oromia, SNNP, Somali and Tigray regions respectively (Gari, 2012).

2.2.3. Host Risk Factor and Susceptibility

Lumpy skin disease is a disease of cattle and causes several disorders. Though all breeds and all age group, both sex are susceptible, Bos *taurus* are particularly more vulnerable to clinical disease than zebu cattle. Among *Bos taurus,* fine-skinned Channel Island breeds develop more severe disease because of their thin skin, although younger animals are usually affecting and show more severe disease than adult ones and Asian water buffalo are also reported to be susceptible (OIE, 2010).

5

Even though, the clinical severity of disease depends on susceptibility and immunological status of the thin-skinned, the high-producing dairy animal *Bos taurus* breeds are highly susceptible against LSDV, whereas indigenous (*Bos indicus*) breeds such as zebu and zebu hybrids are likely to have some natural resistance against the virus (Gari *et al.*, 2011). It is not known what genetic factors influence the disease severity (Babiuk *et al.* 2008).

Lactating cows appearing to be severely affected and result in a sharp drop in milk production because of high fever caused by viral infection itself and secondary bacterial mastitis (Tuppurainen and Oura, 2011). High ambient temperatures, coupled with farming practices to produce high milk yields, could be deemed to stress the animals and contribute to the severity of the disease in Holstein–Friesian cattle (Tageldin *et al.*, 2014). The morbidity rate varies widely depending on the immune status of the hosts (Host susceptibility) and the abundance of mechanical arthropod vectors (CFSPH, 2011). An introduction of new animals to the herd was highly associated with the occurrence of LSD (Birhanu, 2012). There is no evidence or report that the virus can affect humans (OIE, 2011),

2.3.4. Role of Wildlife

In general, CaPVs are highly host specific (Domestic cattle and water buffaloes), with only a few known exceptions some wild species but Role of wildlife still has to be clarified as Giraffe (Giraffe Camelopardalis) and impala (Aepyceros melampus) are highly susceptible to experimental infection. Suspected clinical disease has been described in an Arabian oryx (Oryx leucoryx) in Saudi Arabia, springbok (Antidorcas marsupialis) in Namibia, and oryx (Oryx gazelle) in South Africa and Thomson's gazelle have been infected experimentally by parenteral inoculation with LSDV and have developed characteristic lesions. However, under natural conditions, lesions of LSD have not been seen on these animals when they have been present during epizootics of the disease (Padilla *et al.*, 2005). African buffaloes (*Syncerus caffer*) and Asian water buffaloes (*Bubalus bubalis)* do not show lesions in the field during epizootics of LSD but both buffalo types may suffer an unapparent infection (Tuppurainen, 2015). Thus, the normally the role of wildlife in the transmission and maintenance of LSDV was found almost negligible (Zeynalova *et al.*, 2016).

2.3.5. Environmental Risk Factor

The effect of agroclimate, communal share of the same grazing and watering points and unrestricted movement of animals across different borders following rainfall were some of the risk factors (Tuppurainen and Oura, 2011). Distribution of the disease in various agro climatic conditions, introduction of new animals to the herd and the presence water bodies are among the other risk factors also that would facilitate the spread of outbreaks in various localities (Sameea *et al.*, 2016). The incidence of LSD occurrence is high during wet seasons when biting-fly populations are abundant and it decreases or ceases during the dry season (Gari *et al.*, 2010).

2.3.6. Pathogen Risk Factor

LSDV is generally resistant to drying, survive freezing and thawing. Resistance to heat is variable but most are inactivated at temperatures above 60°C (Radostits *et al.*, 2006). It survives well at cold temperatures (Lefevre and Gourreau, 2010). LSDV is very resistant to physical and chemical agents. The virus persists in necrotic skin for at least 33 days and remains viable in lesions in air-dried hides for at least 18 days at ambient temperature (Vorster and Mapham, 2008). It may persist for up to six months in a suitable environment, such as shaded animal pens. The virus is also present in nasal, lachrymal and pharyngeal secretions, semen, milk and blood and it may remain in saliva for up to 11 days and in semen for 22 days (Annandale, 2014).

There is no evidence of the virus persisting in meat of infected animals, but it might be isolated from milk in early stages of fever (Alaa *et al.*, 2008). The virus may persist for months in lesions in cattle hides. LSD virus may persist for 6 months on fomites, including clothing and equipment but there is no evidence that virus can survive more than four days in insect vectors (Lefevre and Gourreau, 2010).

2.2.7. Mode of transmission

Though there was no clearly defined method of transmission of LSD but the circumstantial evidences suggests that disease might be transmitted by biting insects (Sameea *et al.*, 2016). And now are well-expressed the main mode of transmission of LSDV is *via* arthropod vectors whereas direct or indirect contact between infected and susceptible animals or using contaminated objects or materials by clinically sick animals is an inefficient method of transmission. Subsequently, the virus was isolated from arthropod vectors and the role of vectors in transmission of the virus as experimentally confirmed (Tuppurainen, 2015).

Three bloods sucking hard tick species, *Aedes aegypti* mosquitoes and *Stomoxys calcitrans* flies, have been reported to involve in the transmission of LSDV in sub-Saharan Africa. The three tick species identified as vectors of the disease and also act as 'reservoirs' for the virus are the *Rhipicephalus (Boophilus) decoloratus* (blue tick), *Rhipicephalus appendiculatus* (brown ear tick) and *Amblyomma* hebraeum (bont tick). (Lubinga, 2014).

All secretions of the infected animal virus are present in blood, nasal and lachrymal secretions, semen and saliva, milk, which may be sources for transmission alongside LSD virus when nodules on the mucous membranes of the eyes, nose, mouth, rectum, udder and genitalia ulcerate are also importance source (Babiuk *et al.*, 2008b). Additional, LSD is transmissible to suckling calves through infected milk (Lefèvre and Gourreau, 2010).

Therefore, the main pathways for transmission are biting and blood-feeding arthropods, including biting flies, mosquitoes and ticks. Though rare, transmission also occurs through direct contact, and can also spread from contaminated feed and water (Ali *et al.*, 2012).

2.2.8. Pathogenesis.

During the acute stage of skin lesions, histopathological changes include vasculitis and lymphangitis with concomitant thrombosis and infarction, which result in to oedema and necrosis. LSD skin nodules may exude serum initially but develop a characteristic inverted greyish pink conical zone of necrosis. Adjacent tissue exhibits congestion, haemorrhages and oedema. The necrotic cores become separated from the adjacent skin and are referred to as 'sit-fasts'. Enlarged lymph nodes are found and secondary bacterial infections are common within the necrotic cores. Multiple virus-encoded factors are produced during infection, which influence pathogenesis and disease (Tuppurainen and Oura, 2012).

3. Clinical signs and postmortem lesion

The disease is characterized by large skin nodules covering all parts of the body, fever, enlarged lymph nodes, loss of appetite, reduction in milk production, some depression and reluctance to move nasal discharge and lachrymation. Young calves often have more severe disease than adults (CFSPH, 2011). The severity of clinical signs of LSD depends on the host immunity status, age, sex and breed type. The more susceptible breeds to LSD infection are related to fine-skinned breeds such as Holstein Friesian (HF) and Jersey breeds (Kumar, 2011). Additional, the disease affects cattle and tends to be more severe in milking cows in the peak of lactation as a result of mastitis, was suffered by a number of dairy farmers as well in young animals (Gari *et al.*, 2011).

Lumpy skin disease may be occur acute, sub-acute and chronic forms (OIE, 2010). It has an incubation period of 2 to 4 weeks in the field (Tuppurainen and Oura, 2012). The nodules developed on skin are vary from 2 cm to 7 cm in diameter, appearing as round, well circumscribed areas of erect hair, firm and slightly raised from the surrounding skin and particularly conspicuous in short-haired animals. In long-haired cattle the nodules are often only recognized when the skin is palpated or moistened. In most cases the nodules are particularly noticeable in the hairless areas of perineum, udder, inner ear, muzzle, eyelids and on the vulva. Alongside other common sites are head and neck, genitalia, limb and udder; involve skin, cutaneous tissues, legs and some time underlying part of the muscle (Alemayehu *et al.,* 2013).

Histopathology can be an important tool to exclude viral, bacterial or fungal causes of nodular development in clinical cases and characteristic cytopathic effects (necrosed epidermis, ballooning degeneration of squamous epithelialcells and eosinophilic intracytoplasmic inclusion bodies) in cases of lumpy skin disease are well documented (Brenner *et al.*, 2006). Lesion of lumpy skin diseases showed presence of eosinophilic intracytoplasmic inclusions bodies was easily recorded due to lumpy skin disease virus (Tuppurainen *et al.*, 2011).

3.1. Diagnosis

Field diagnosis of LSD is often based on characteristic clinical signs of the disease. However, mild and subclinical forms require rapid and reliable laboratory testing to confirm diagnosis (Alaa *et al.*, 2008). Most commonly used methods of diagnosing LSD are detecting virus DNA using the polymerase chain reaction (PCR), Different molecular tests are also the preferred diagnostic tools or by detecting antibodies to LSD virus using serology-based diagnostic tests (OIE, 2010). Rapid diagnostic confirmation of the tentative field diagnosis is fundamental for the successful control and eradication of LSD in endemic and particularly in non-endemic countries (EFSA Journal, 2015). In addition Laboratory test of LSD can be made by identification of the agent, routine histopathological examination and immune histological staining (Tuppurainen, 2011).

3.2. Differential diagnosis

Although severe LSD is highly characteristic, but milder forms can be confused and misdiagnosed with numerous skin diseases of cattle that could be considered as differential diagnosis are: Bovine Herpes Mammilitis (Pseudo-lumpy skin disease): The presence of Bovine Herpes Mammilitis case has not yet been confirmed by laboratory in Ethiopia. Dermatophilosis: *Dermatophilus congolensis* infection is one of wide spread skin disease of cattle in Ethiopia and lesions could be differentiated from LSD in that the lesions of Dermatophilosis are superficial (often moist and appear as crusts of keratinized material) scabs of 0.5- to 2 cm diameter. The organism can be demonstrated by Giemsa staining. Demodicosis, Besnoitiosis, Photosensitization, insect bites; and Ringworm could also be considered as the differential diagnosis. Epidemiological features could help to distinguish LSD vs. other skin lesions (OIE, 2009). A definitive diagnosis can only be confirmed by submitting appropriate samples of skin lesions to a laboratory where the virus can be identified. Molecular diagnostic tests such as conventional and real-time polymerase chain reaction (PCR) assays are rapid and highly sensitive tests, and are widely used in veterinary diagnostic laboratories (EFSA Journal, 2015).

3.3. Occurrence and Current Status of Lumpy Skin Disease in Ethiopia.

As Ethiopia has the largest number of livestock population in Africa. The Ethiopian economy is highly dependent on agriculture, which contributed about 48% of the GDP, followed by 39% from the service sector and 13% from the industrial sector. As a result of the country has much gain from the growing global market for livestock products. However, the livestock disease is one of the major livestock production constraints including LSD. LSD is one of the newly emerging diseases of cattle in Ethiopia. (Gebreegziabhare, 2010). The current status and occurrence of LSD is associate with the different agro-climatic conditions and the associated risk factors. There are three variables expected to influence the distribution and occurrence of LSD in Ethiopia: the effect of agro climate, communal grazing/watering management and introduction of new animals. Moreover, Ethiopia has two major seasons of rainfall: a shorter rainy season that usually begins in mid-February and continues up to end of April and the long rainy season (75%) starting mid-June and ending mid September. (Alemayehu, 2009). Hence this association might be attributed to the availability and abundance of effective mechanical vector insects (Fig 3). Thus the temporal involvement between LSD occurrence and increase in the biting-fly population was positively correlated and significant increase to the occurrence of the disease. Consequently both biting-flies activity and disease outbreak frequencies begin to increase from April reaching a maximum in September which suggested that mechanical vector insects might play a major role in the disease outbreak of LSD (Fig 4).

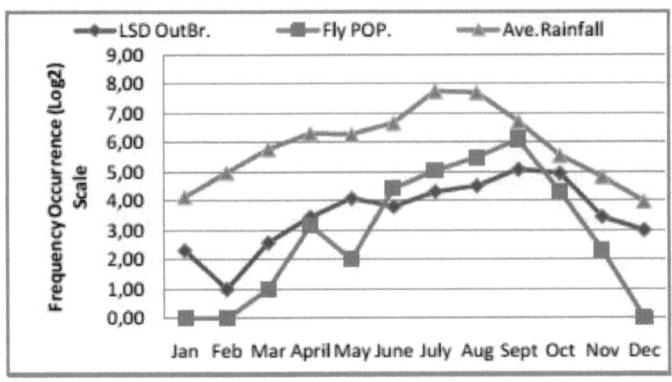

Figure 3: Seasonal increase in biting-fly activity vs. lumpy skin disease (LSD) occurrence (s). Source: (Troyo *et al.*, 2007).

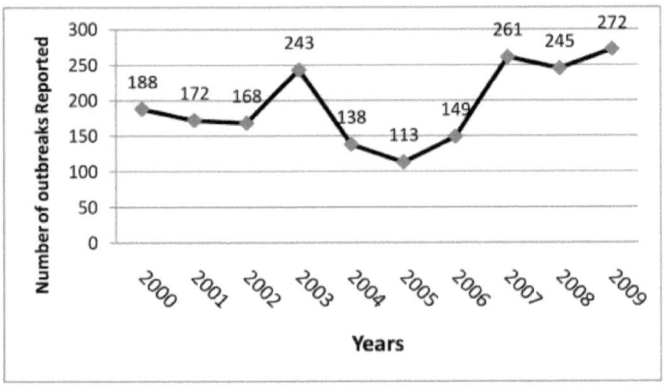

Figure 4: Biting fly population density through the year in 2008/2009 based on fly catchment. Source: Waret-Szkuta *et al.*, 2010).

As mention environmental factor of sharing common watering points and grazing plots would allow contact and intermingling of different herds that would probably increase the risk of exposure and enhance the virus transmission through contamination and/or the speculated mechanical vectors such as Stomoxys spp. and mosquitoes (Waret-Szkuta et al., 2010).

Subsequently the potential risk of agro-climate variations to LSD occurrence showed that herds in midland and lowland agro-climates were more likely infected by LSD than in the highland agro-climate. Seeing that the herd level sero-prevalence was higher in the midland (64 %) as compared to the lowland (50 %) and the highland (26 %) (Abera *et al.*, 2015) because Agro-climate variation is the basis for the type and abundance of considered mechanical vector insects. Therefore, the warm and humid climate in midland agro-climates might be a more favorable environment for the occurrence of large populations of biting flies than the remaining two agro-climates (Tiwari *et al.*, 2009) (Fig. 5).

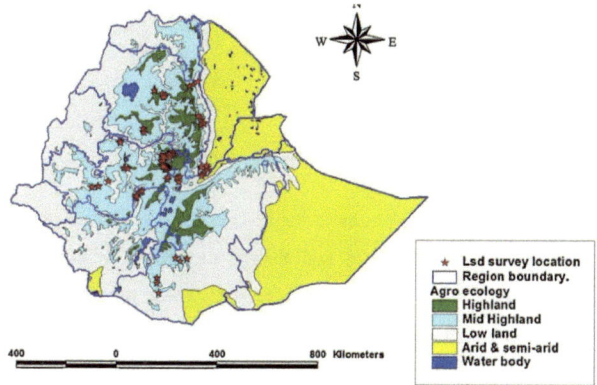

Figure 5: LSD locations and major agro-climate zones in Ethiopia. Source (Abera, 2015).

As shown in Table 1 below in Ethiopia in 2007-2011 total of 1352 diseases outbreak of LSD has been reported. The highest disease outbreaked was documented in Oromiya region and the least in Afar region.

Table 1: As regards Reported outbreaks and LSD affected populations in different regions of Ethiopia from 2007-2011 (Source: Birhanu, 2012).

Zone	Years of reported outbreaks					
	2007	2008	2009	2010	2011	Total
Addis Ababa			3	7	1	11
Afar			3	2	2	7
Amhara	92	68	35	40	22	257
Ben.Gumuz	3				5	8
Gambela				1	9	10
Oromiya	95	154	219	286	160	896
SNNP	18	18	14	32	17	99
Somali			3	9	4	16
Tigray	7	8	2	18	13	48
Grand Total	**215**	**248**	**279**	**377**	**233**	**1352**

3.4. Control and prevention

Till this moment, no specific antiviral treatment for LSD infection has been found. Sick animals should be removed from the herd and follow supportive treatment such as antibiotics, anti-inflammatory drugs, and vitamin injections. These therapies are usually the chances for the development of secondary bacterial infections, inflammation and fever, and thus improving the appetite of the animal (Tuppurainen and Oura, 2012).

Prevention and control of LSD is undertaken through vaccination, quarantines, livestock movement, and control of insect vectors in the initial stages of an outbreak, to minimize mechanical transmission of the virus vector control, slaughter of infected and exposed animals and cleaning and disinfection of the premises, awareness campaign to facilitate cooperation from the industry and the community (Radostits et al., 2006). The biting flies and certain tick species are probably the most important method of transmission of the disease, control by quarantine and movement control is generally not very effective. In endemic areas, control is therefore essentially confined to vaccination or immunoprophylaxis (Rushton, 2009).

Only live attenuated vaccines against LSD are currently commercially available. Live vaccines help control losses from lumpy skin disease in endemic areas. Homologous LSD vaccines are more successful than vaccines based on attenuated sheep pox viruses. Heterologous live attenuated virus vaccine may cause local and sometimes severe reactions. This vaccine is not advised in countries free from sheep and goat pox because the live vaccines could otherwise provide a source of infection for the susceptible sheep and goat populations (Al-Salihi, 2014). Therefore, vaccination is the only successful manner to control the disease in endemic countries but in non-endemic areas, the use of live attenuated vaccines would be highly questionable on the grounds of safety (OIE, 2010).

3.6. Public health

LSD poses no zoonotic problems. Infected cattle are a not a source of any infection for humans and milk is safe to enter the human food chain. Whilst it is not desirable to eat the flesh of infected animals, due to the likelihood of carcass contamination by secondary bacterial infections, no harm has been known to have resulted from its consumption. Hence, there is no evidence and description that the virus can affect humans (Rich and Perry, 2010).

4. Economic impact of the disease

Capri pox viruses are becoming an emerging worldwide threat to sheep, goats and cattle (Babiuk et al., 2008). LSD causes considerable economic losses due to emaciation, hide damage, temporary or permanent infertility in males and females, abortion, mastitis, loss of milk production and mortality of up to 40%, although mortality rarely exceeds 3% (Tuppurainen and Oura 2011). Therefore, Lumpy skin disease is one of the economically significant diseases in Africa and the Middle East countries that cause severe production loss in cattle. The world organization for animal health (OIE) categorizes the disease as notifiable diseases because of its severe economic losses. The economic importance of

15

the disease was mainly due to having high morbidity rate rather than mortality (Tuppurainen and Oura, 2011).

As a consequence the financial implication of these losses is greatly significant to the herd owners, consumers and the industrial sectors which can process the livestock products and by products. Reports from Ethiopia indicated that the financial loss estimated based on milk, meat, beef, draught power, mortality, treatment and vaccination costs in individual head of local zebu were lost 6.43 USD and for the Holstein Friesian 58 USD (Getachew *et al.*, 2010).

In general LSD is considered as a disease of high economic pressure because of its ability to compromise food security through loss, draft power, reduced output of animal production, increase production costs due to increased costs of disease control, and disrupt livestock and their product trade. Moreover, severe economic losses may be high due to condemnation of carcass and cost of inspecting meat as it damage to the hides (Kumar, 2011). Permanent damage to the skin and hide greatly affect leather industry. It causes ban on international trade of livestock and causes prolonged economic loss as it became endemic and brought serious stock loss. Restrictions to the global trade of live animals and animal products, costly control and eradication measures such as vaccination campaigns as well as the indirect costs because of the compulsory limitations in animal movements cause significant financial losses on a national level (Alkhamis and VanderWaal, 2016).

5. CONCLUSION AND RECOMMENDATION

Lumpy skin disease (LSD) is a generalized skin disease which is an infectious, eruptive, occasionally fatal disease of cattle caused by a virus associated with the Neethling poxvirus in the genus Capri poxvirus of the family Poxviridae. LSD was first described in Zambia and occurs in other most African countries and currently endemic in most African countries and has recently spread out of Africa into the Middle East regions, Asia and Europe. In Ethiopia, LSD was first observed in 1983 in the north-western part of the country (south-west of Lake Tana). Mechanical vector of arthropods play main role in transmission of the virus while wildlife a plays role as a reservoir for LSDV outbreaks with typically associated with wet and warm seasons. Pathogen, environment and host factors are considered as main risk factors for the disease. The severity of clinical sign of LSD may be acute or sub acute form which depends on cattle breeds, ages and sexes factors. The disease is more severe in young animals and cows in the peak of lactation. LSD can be diagnosed using appropriate serological and molecular techniques. The disease can result in economic limitations to the global trade of live animals and animal products. The control of LSD can be achieved through vaccination, restriction of animal movement and eradication of infected and exposed animals. Based on the above conclusion the following recommendations are forwarded.

- ❖ The government should establish strategic policies for effective control and eradication of the disease, i.e. restriction of livestock movement, strategic vaccination program and depopulation of infected and in contact animals.
- ❖ Further research is required to elucidate vector insects incriminated in the transmission of LSDV and their dynamics in different agro-ecologies.
- ❖ Implementation of quarantine system before new animals introduced to the herd.
- ❖ Regular community knowledge that the herd owners should avoid herd mixing and contacts by using private grazing plots and watering sources.
- ❖ To develop the main method to control LSD is through Ring and mass vaccination cattle.

6. REFERENCES

Abera, Z., Degefu, H., Gari, G. and Kidane, M. (2015). Sero-prevalence of lumpy skin disease in selected districts of West Wollega zone, Ethiopia. *Biomedical Center of veterinary research,* **11**:135.

Ahmed, W. & Kawther, S. (2008). Observations on lumpy skin disease in local Egyptian cows with emphasis on its impact on ovarian function. *Africa. Journal. Microbiology Research,* **2**: 252–257.

Alaa, A., Hatem, M., Khaled A. (2008). Polymerase chain reaction for rapid diagnosis of a recent lumpy skin disease virus incursion to *Egypt. Journal. Arabian Biotechnology,* **11**:293-302.

Alemayehu, G., Zewde, G., and Admassu, B. (2013). Risk assessments of lumpy skin diseases in borena bull market chain and it implication for livelihoods and international trade. *Tropical. Animal. Health Production,* **45:** 1153–1159.

Alemayehu, M. (2009). Country pasture/ forage profiles; http://www.fao.org/ag/AGP/AGPC/doc/pasture/forage.htm. (Accessed: February 22, 2017).

Ali, H., Ali, A., Atta, M.S. & Cepica, A. (2012). Common, emerging, vector-borne and infrequent abortogenic virus infections of cattle. *Transbound Emerge Diseases,* **59**: 11–25.

Alkhamis, M.A. and VanderWaal, K. (2016). Spatial and Temporal epidemiology of lumpy skin Disease in the Middle east, 2012–2015. *Frontiers in veterinary science,* **3**.44-52.

Al-Salihi, K. A. (2014). Lumpy Skin disease: Review of literature. *Mirror Research. Veterinary,* **3**: 6-23.

Annandale, C.H., Holm, D.E., Ebersohn, K. and Venter, E.H. (2014). Seminal transmission of lumpy skin disease virus in heifers. *Transboundary and emerging diseases,* **61**: 443-448.

18

Annandale, C.H., Irons, P.C. Bagla, V.P., Osuagwuh, U.I. and Venter, E.H. (2010). Sites of persistence of lumpy skin disease virus in the genital tract of experimentally infected bulls. *Reproduction in domestic animals*, **45**: 250-255.

Anon. (2009). Export products of Ethiopia in all regions; (http://www.addismillennium.com/majorexportproductsofethiopia2.htm).(Accessed January 27, 2017).

Babiuk, S., Bowden, T., Boyle, D., Wallace, D., Kitching, R.P. (2008b). Capripoxviruses: an emerging world¬wide threat to sheep goats and cattle. *Transboundary and Emerging Diseases*, **55**: 263-272.

Babiuk, S., T.R. Bowden, D.B. Boyle, D.B. Wallace, and R.P. Kitching. (2008). Capripoxviruses: an emerging worldwide threat to sheep, goats and cattle. *Transboundary. Emergency. Diseases*. **55**: 263–272

Bagla, V.P. (2008). The demonstration of lumpy skin disease virus in semen of experimentally infected bulls using different diagnostic techniques (Doctoral dissertation).Pp.76-84.

Birhanu. (2012). Assessments of the risk factors and financial impacts of LSD in selected districts of Tigray and Afar Regional States, Northeastern Ethiopia M.Sc. Thesis.Pp.24-33.

Brenner, J., Haimovitz, M., Orone E., Stram Y., Fridgut O., Bumbarov V., Kuznetzova, L., Oved Z., Waerrman A., Garazzi S., Perl S., Lahav D., Edery N. &Yadin H. (2006). Lumpy skin disease (LSD) in a large dairy herd in Israel. *Israel. Journal. Veterinary. Medicine*, **61**:73–77.

CFSPH. (2008). The Center for Food Security and Public Health, Iowa State University, College of Veterinary Medicine and Institution of International cooperation in Animal Biologics, an OIE collaborating center.

CFSPH. (2011). Center for Food Security and Public Health, Iowa State University, 2011 College of Veterinary Medicine.Pp.55-67.

CSA (Central Statistical Agency). (2016). Report on livestock and livestock characteristics. Vol II, Statistical Bulletin. P.583.

Efsa, N. D. A. (2015). Panel (EFSA Panel on Dietetic Products, Nutrition and Allergies). *Scientific opinion on dietary reference values for vitamin. Journal*, **13**: 4028-4084.

FAO. (2009). Livestock in balance. Food and Agriculture Organization of the United Nations, Vialedelleterme di Caracalla 00153 Rome, Italy (http://www.fao.org/nr/water/). (Accessed March 1, 2017).

FAO. (2009). Livestock in balance. Food and Agriculture Organization of the United Nations, Vialedelleterme di Caracalla 00153 Rome, Italy.P.23.

Gari, G., A.Waret-Szkuta, V.Grosbois, P.Jacquiet and considered. F. Roger. (2010). Risk factors associated with observed clinical lumpy skin disease in Ethiopia. *Epidemiology. Infection*, **138**:1657-1666.

Gari, G., Bonnet, P., Roger, F., Waret-Szkuta, A. (2011). Epidemiological aspects and financial impact of lumpy skin disease in Ethiopia. *Preventive. Veterinary. Medicine*, **102**: 274– 283.

Gari, G., Grosbois, V., Waret-Szkuta, A., Babiuk, S., Jacquiet, P. and Roger, F. (2012). Lumpy skin disease in Ethiopia: Seroprevalence study across different agro-climate zones. *Acta tropical*, **123**: 101-106.

Gebreegziabhare, B. (2010). An over view of the role of Ethiopian livestock in livelihood and Food safety. Ministry of Agriculture and Rural development of Ethiopia; Presente on dialogue on livestock, food security and sustainability, a side event on the session of 22 COAGO, FAO, Rome.Pp. 581-593.

Getachew, G., Waret-Szkuta, A., Grosbois, V., andJacquite, P. (2010). Risk Factors Associated with observed clinical lumpy skin disease in Ethiopia. PhD thesis. Pp.68-84.

Gelaye, E., Belay, A., Ayelet, G., Jenberie, S., Yami, M., Loitsch, A., Tuppurainen, E., Grabherr, R., Diallo, A. and Lamien, C.E. (2015). Capripox disease in Ethiopia: genetic differences between field isolates and vaccine strain, and implications for vaccination failure. *Antiviral research*, **119**: 28-35.

J. Brenner. (2006). "Lumpy skin disease (LSD) in a large dairy herd in Israel," *Israel. Journal. Veterinary. Medicine*, **61**: 73-77.

Kumar, S.M. (2011). An outbreak of lumpy skin disease in a Holstein dairy herd in Oman: a clinical report. *Asian Journal of Animal and Veterinary Advances*, **6**: 851-859.

Lefèvre, P.C., Gourreau, J.M. (2010). Lumpy Skin disease. In: Lefèvre, P.C., Blancou, J., Chermette, R., Uilenberg, G. (Eds.), Infectious and Parasitic diseases of Livestock. Lavoisier, Paris, 393-407.

Lubinga, J.C., Clift, E.S., Tuppurainen, W.H., Stoltsz, S.B., Abiuk, J.A., Coetze.r and Venter, E.H. (2014). Demonstration of lumpy skin disease virus infectionin *Amblyomma hebraeum and Rhipicephalusappendiculatus* ticks using immunohistochemistry. *Ticks Tick Borne Diseases*, **5**: 113-20.

Mebratu, G.Y., B. Kassa, Y. Fikre. and B. Bethany. (1984). Observations on the outbreak of lumpy skin disease in Ethiopia. La Revue d'Elevage et de Médecine Vétérinaire des Pays Tropicaux, 37: 395-399.

OIE. (2008). Lumpy skin disease. In: Manual of Diagnostic Tests and Vaccines for Terrestrial Animals. Office International des Epizooties, World Organization for Animal Health, Paris. Pp. 768 -779.

OIE. (2009). Lumpy Skin Disease. Etiology, Epidemiology, Diagnosis, Prevention and Control References. Terrestrial Animal Health Code. OIE, Paris. **3**:127 -135.

OIE. (2010). OIE Manual of Diagnostic Tests and Vaccines for Terrestrial Animals .Lumpy skin disease.Chapter2.4.14. Pp.768-778.

OIE. (2010). Terrestrial Manual of Lumpy Skin Disease, Chapter 2.4.14. Version adopted by the World Assembly of Delegates of the OIE. Paris. Pp.425-431.

OIE. (2011). Lumpy Skin Disease. Terrestrial Animal Health Code. OIE, Paris. Pp.268-276.

OIE. (2015b). Lumpy skin disease – Greece. Date of start of event 18/08/2015. Available at: http://www.oie.int/wahis_2/public/wahid.php/. (Accessed February 23, 2017).

Padilla, L.R., Dutton, C.J., Bauman, J. and Duncan, M. (2005). XY male pseudohermaphroditism in a captive Arabian oryx (Oryx leucoryx). *Journal of zoo and wildlife medicine*, **36**: 498-503.

Radostits, M., Gay, C., Hinchcliff, W., Constable, D. (2006). Veterinary medicine A text book of the diseases of cattle, horses, sheep, pigs and goats 10th ed. WB Saunders Co., Philadelphia, USA, Pp. 1424- 1426.

RGBE, H. (2014). Lumpy skin disease (LSD): outbreak investigation, isolation and molecular detection of lumpy skin disease in selected areas of eastern Shewa, Ethiopia (Doctoral dissertation, AAU).P.72.

Rich, K.M. and Perry, B.D. (2010). The economic and poverty impacts of animal diseases indeveloping countries: New roles, new demands for economics and epidemiology. *Preentive. Veterinary. Medicine.***6**.142-161.

Rushton, J. and Leonard, D. K. (2009). 12 The New Institutional Economics and the Assessment of Animal Disease Control. *The Economics of Animal Health and Production,* **4**.144.

Sajid, A., Chaudhary, Z., Sadique, U., Maqbol, A., Anjum, A., Qureshi, M. (2012). Prevalence of goat pox disease in Punjab province of Pakistan. *Journal. Animal. Plant Science.* **22**: 28–32.

Salib, F.A. and Osman, A.H. (2011). Incidence of lumpy skin disease among Egyptian cattle in Giza Governorate, Egypt. *Veterinary World,* **4**:162-167.

Sameea, Yousefi, P., Mardani, K., Dalir, Naghadeh, B. and Jalilzadeh-Amin, G. (2016). Epidemiological Study of Lumpy Skin Disease Outbreaks in North - western Iran. *Transboundary and Emerging Diseases*. **3**:109-117.

Tageldin, M.H., Wallace, D.B., Gerdes, G.H., Putterill, J.F., Greyling, R.R., Phosiwa, M.N., Al-Busaidy, R.M. and Al-Ismaaily, S.I. (2014). Lumpy skin disease of cattle: an emerging problem in the Sultanate of Oman. Tropical *animal health and production*, **46**: 241-246.

Troyo, A., Calderon-Arguedas, O., Fuller, D.O., Solano, M.E., Avendano, A., Arheart, K.L., Chadee, D.D., Beier, J.C. (2007). Seasonal profiles of Aedes aegypti (Diptera: Culicidae) Larval habitats in an urban area of Costa Rica with the history of mosquito control. *Journal of Vector Ecology* **33**: 1-13.

Thornton, P.K. (2010). Livestock production: recent trends, future prospects. *The Royal Society*, **365**:2853-2867.

Tiwari, A., VanLeeuwen, J.A., Dohoo, I.R., Keefe, G.P., Haddad, J.P., Scott, H.M., Whiting, T. (2009). Risk factors associated with Myco¬bacterium avium subspecies paratuberculosis sero¬positivity in Canadian dairy cows and herds. *Preventive. Veterinary. Medicine,* **88**: 32-41.

Tschopp, R., Schelling, E., Hattendorf, J., Aseffa, A., Zinsstag, J. (2009). Risk factors of bovine tuberculosis in cattle in rural livestock production systems of Ethiopia. *Preventive. Veterinary. Medicine,* **89**: 205-211.

Tuppurainen, E. (2015). Evaluation of vector potential of *Rhipicephalus appendiculatus, Amblyomma hebraeum and Rhipicephalus decoloratus ticks for lumpy skin disease virus.* **13**: 225-231.

Tuppurainen, E. S. M. and Oura. C. A. L. (2011). Review: Lumpy Skin Disease: An Emerging Threat to Europe, the Middle East and Asia, *Institute for Animal Health, Pirbright, and Surrey, United Kingdom.6:* 243-255.

Tuppurainen, E.S.M., Oura, C.A.L. (2012). Review: lumpy skin disease: an emerging threat to Europe, the Middle East and Asia. *Transbound. Emerge. Diseases*, **59**:40–48.

Tuppurainen, S. M. (2005). Detection of the lumpy skin disease virus in samples of the experimentally infected cattle using different diagnostic techniques, MSc thesis.Pp.15-22.

Vorster, H., Mapham, H. (2008). Pathology of lumpy skin disease. Livestock Health and *Production Review*, **1**:16-21.

Waret-Szkuta, A., Ortiz-Pelaez, A., Roger, F., Pfeiffer, D.U., Guitian, F.J. (2010). Herd contact structure based on shared use of water points and grazing points in the Highlands of Ethiopia. *Epidemiology. Infection.* **11**: 235-241.

Yehuda, S., Larisa, O., Boris G., Hagai, Y., Marisol, R. (2011). The use of lumpy skin disease virus genome termini for detection and phylogenetic analysis. *Journal. Virological Methods*, **151**: 225–229.

Zeynalova, S., Asadov, K., Guliyev, F., Vatani, M. and Aliyev, V. (2016). Epizootology and molecular diagnosis of lumpy skin disease among livestock in Azerbaijan. *Frontiers in Microbiology*, **8.** 271.

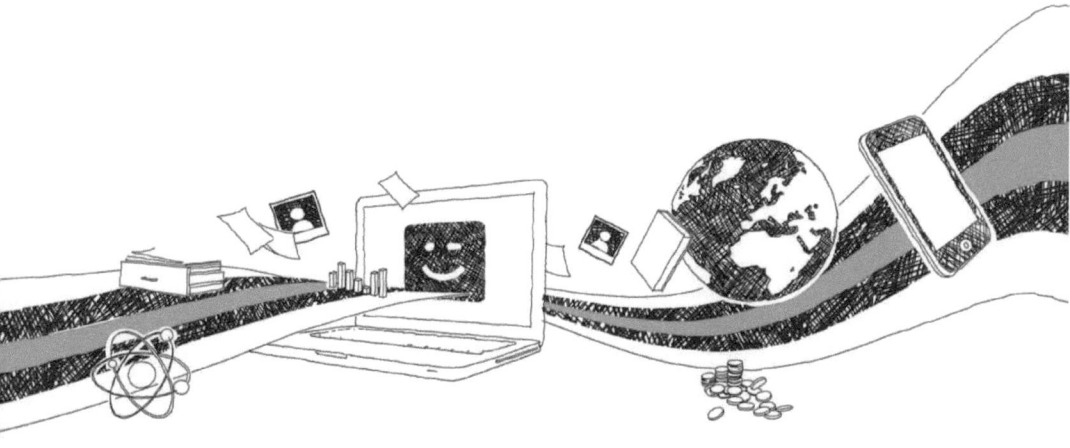
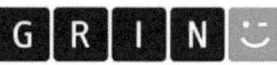